Exercises for Seeing Mindfully Volume One

Mindfulness Practices for Persons with Parkinson's Disease

9/3/2014
Parkinsons Recovery
Robert Rodgers PhD

Contents

The Parkinsons Recovery Mindfulness Series

Realistically speaking, how can the intense level of stress that aggravates the symptoms of Parkinson's disease be calmed? Better yet, how can they be quieted? My research over the past decade reveals that using your mind to drop the stress level down a notch or two always backfires. When you tell yourself:

- *Settle down!*
- *Take it easy!*
- *Stop being so stressed out!*

The stress level ratchets up, not down. Attempts to force the stress and anxiety levels to adjust downward induce an internally generated stress. They pile more stress on top of an excess of stress that already exists. There are certainly a sufficient number of external generators of stress in every one's life. Why infuse more stress that you create yourself, even with the best of intentions?

If the mind is not a useful technique to reduce stress, what is? The most eloquent answer I have for you is to become more mindful of what is experienced in the present moment. Becoming more mindful shifts you into the experience of the "now" which in itself is less stressful (unless you have been kidnapped by terrorists!).

It is stressful to anticipate events you imagine will occur in the future. The events we imagine rarely happen. Does this ring true for you? We all create unnecessary stress in our lives by how and where we focus our thoughts and attention.

It is stressful to agonize over the past. When we think about the past, we are much more likely to think about unpleasant experiences that induce stress. The past event itself was traumatic enough. Yet, we insist on reliving the trauma over and over again through our memories. It seems some of us just can't get enough stress in our lives.

The problem with upping the ante on stress levels is that – as you well know – symptoms of Parkinson's disease become worse. When you are not as stressed, your symptoms are far less problematic.

I have reached one solid conclusion from my ten years of research on Parkinson's disease. Symptoms will drive you crazy when you are stressed and are far less problematic when stress is under control.

Now, if you can't use your mind to become more mindful (which creates added stress in itself) how in the world can you quiet down a frantic lifestyle? I have concluded that the simplest and most effective solution to reducing stress levels is to become more mindful.

The transformation is possible step by step through these simple exercises you can do anywhere, anytime of the day. The Parkinsons Recovery mindfulness exercises are designed to focus your attention on the present moment as attention on either the past or the future is diverted. A renewed focus on the present moment reduces stress levels. Mindfulness is a lifestyle that will reduce stresses in your life if you set the intention to take a mindfulness practice seriously.

I recommend that you practice each of the exercises for a week or longer. Incorporate each practice into your regular routines and habits. Attempts to do all of the exercises simultaneously will likely induce more stress which – obviously – is contrary to the intent of a successful mindfulness program.

Give each exercise a little time and space. Invite the stresses in your life to dissipate. Allow the experience of each practice to engulf you. In so doing, watch the stresses in your life dip down to new lows along with a concurrent relief of any and all symptoms that you have currently been experiencing.

This volume is one out of nine I have developed to support the recovery of persons who currently experience neurological symptoms. A full listing of the Parkinsons Recovery Mindfulness booklets follows:

Exercises for Seeing Mindfully
Mindfulness Practices for Persons with Parkinson's Disease
Volume One

Robert Rodgers, PhD

Parkinsons Recovery

www.parkinsonsrecovery.me

Olympia, Washington

Exercise One: Vision Quest

You are cordially invited to pursue a Vision Quest this week. What in the world do I mean by a Vision Quest? The Vision Quest I propose is not about going out into the forest and sitting in a circle for four days without food or water. So, stay with me on this one. The Vision Quest I have in mind is actually simple to do, yet profound.

The Vision Quest that I propose for you to explore was inspired by Darlene Cohen who is a well-known author and an expert in helping individuals cope with chronic illness. Darlene suggested in an interview that I did with her several years ago that one of the ways she was successfully able to cope with her chronic illness was to take in the full senses wherever she happened to be. She would look at and take in every detail that she could find in whatever place she happened to find herself. This, as it turned out, expanded her awareness. It helped her become more mindful of being present in the moment. Whatever physical discomfort in the physical body might have been present simply fades away into the sunset.

The Vision Quest is very simply designed and simple to do. It can potentially have profound implications on your ability to maintain centeredness and balance and on your ability moment-to-moment to maintain a stress-free body.

The Vision Quest Challenge

Whenever you sit down – and it does not matter where you sit – the challenge is to look around from wherever you are sitting and find something that you have not noticed before and look at it. Take in its full essence. That is it folks.

We get accustomed to our routines. We walk from our bedroom as we are getting up to the kitchen. Many of us prepare either a cup of hot tea or coffee and then we sit down at a table, at a chair or perhaps in front of our computer or television. We do not really look anywhere because out routine is so habitual. We do not take in the beauty and nuances of our environment. Our minds are somewhere else. Our body simply runs through a rat maze day after day, missing all the beauty that surrounds us.

The challenge is to expand your awareness through sight. Every time you sit down, trigger an awareness that says,

> *"Wait. I just found myself sitting down. I'm now going to look around where I am at and find something that perhaps I really haven't noticed before. Or, if I've noticed everything that I see here where I am sitting, let me really intensely look at something that I haven't taken the opportunity to appreciate."*

7

Expanding awareness through greater vision is one of the powerful techniques for becoming more mindful, more centered, more aware in the moment and more grounded.

Every time you sit down, immediately look to see something you haven't noticed before. You may spend only five or ten seconds looking. You may spend several minutes or perhaps even longer taking in the texture, the color and the essence of what you are looking at.

Break out of the hamster wheel routine of how you normally sense the world that surrounds you. When you sit, set into motion a new way of presenting yourself to the world. Allow its essence to penetrate every cell of your body. Look at familiar objects and sights with fresh eyes.

Enjoy your vision quest however you wish to proceed. Each time you sit, find something new to notice. Stay focused on the purpose here: When stress is eliminated, symptoms wither away.

Deeper Meaning Behind a Vision Quest

We have certainly all discovered in our personal lives the incredible value of focus and the incredible value of setting goals. It works.

- *When we get up in the day ...*
- *When we have a clear vision of exactly what we want to accomplish that day ...*

- *When we have a very specific plan …*

We are able to implement this plan and by the end of the day it is done. Finished. We can accomplish precisely the goal that we established the first thing in the morning.

When we do this day after day and when we have an overall vision of where we are headed, we become very successful individuals. Focus works. It succeeds. It allows us to make miracles happen in our lives.

There is however, a formidable downside to focus. With focus we narrow mindedly center on a very tiny aspect of what it means to be alive, of what it means to feel the full pleasure of occupying a body. One of the serious consequences of focus is that we pump out our adrenaline minute after minute. Our bodies never have the opportunity to settle into that delicious state of relaxation. When our bodies are pumping out adrenaline continuously, it is no wonder that after a few years our hormones are completely whacked. It is no wonder that the body says,

> *"Hey, there's no real need or necessity for me to manufacture any dopamine because this body isn't asking for it and doesn't need it."*

Of course, without dopamine our bodies suffer serious neurological implications.

The idea of a vision quest as an exercise – and I might say, a very simple exercise at that – is to invite you to acknowledge and honor the value of focus but concurrently recognize how that has constrained the experience of living life to its fullest. Open up a vision of seeing what is missed from moment to moment. Lo and behold - you begin to take in the full pleasures, the full wonders of what the world has to offer. When we focus our awareness on the miracles of the moment, our 40 or so hormones are invited to come back into full balance and harmony.

A vision quest then is an invitation to open up a narrow focus wider and wider and wider each time you sit; so that-

- By the end of the week
- By the end of the month
- By the end of the year

You make it habit to take in with your vision the deliciousness of what it means to be present to your world in a fully occupied body.

You can still focus. You can still set goals. But at the same time, it is possible to open up your vision of what you are seeing moment-to-moment. The vision quest is most successful when you are in environments that are totally familiar.

There will be pictures that you hung years ago that you actually haven't looked at or taken in for perhaps decades. Do that now.

There are items - perhaps knickknacks - in the room where you are sitting now. Notice their eloquence and detail today. Appreciate them in a new way.

Outside there are birds and critters that you may seldom stop to observe or even notice. Notice them now. Observe their beauty.

Notice how your body immediately settles into a place of deep relaxation.

The symptoms of Parkinson's are no longer able to rear their ugly head when stress is not present. Bringing yourself into a place of centeredness and balance moment to moment means that stress cannot be a part of who you are in that moment.

To summarize, each time you sit down

1. Find something new to look at.
2. Take the image in fully and completely.
3. Enjoy the deliciousness of what it means to be alive and in a physical body.

Exercise Two: Celebrate Light

I invite you to extend all considerations of where light shines in your life. Acknowledge, notice, honor and celebrate light which is a resource that we all take for granted. When you see sunshine, celebrate the rays of sun as they pass through the leaves of trees. Celebrate the feeling on your skin as the sun touches your body. The sun is a genuine and authentic source of light. Without it none of us would be alive.

It is also been shown in research studies that individuals who currently experience a neurological challenge associated with the diagnosis of Parkinson's disease are seriously deficient in vitamin D3. D3 is a source that is available through the sun. You can acquire D3 in supplement form, but the authentic source comes from direct exposure to sunshine. Individuals who live in the northwest section of the United States and Canada where there is not as much sun as you find typically in other areas (such as the southern states of the United States) are seriously deficient in vitamin D3. Whether you live in the northwest or the south, when you see the sunshine, celebrate its true magical powers. I say once again, without that presence of the sun none of us would be here today.

Extend your appreciation and acknowledgement and celebration of light beyond simply the natural source which is sunshine.

- *Notice when anyone turns on a light switch or turns it off.*
- *Appreciate what happens when light becomes available in a darkened room.*
- *Acknowledge the headlights of other cars as they are turned on in the evening.*
- *Give thanks to the light from your own headlights which enable you to see when you drive.*
- *Celebrate the light that emanates from fireplaces.*

Recognize all sources of light. Consider the source of that light and all of the individuals who were responsible for making that light become available to you as electricity including the individuals who manufactured the power lines and the individuals who installed the power lines.

Give thanks to all the persons who made possible the energy you experience whether it comes from solar or water or coal. However your power is generated, honor all of the individuals that were responsible as well as the plants and the animals on this earth that contributed to, for example the manufacture and the creation of coal and oil which was actually created millions and millions and millions of years ago.

Notice the light that is also present in darkness for even in darkness there are faint shades of light. In summary, celebrate what we all take for granted—the presence of light in your life. .

Deeper Meaning Behind Light

The deeper meaning behind noticing, acknowledging and honoring all sources of light in your life is actually profound. All humans are light beings. Many people are unaware that all objects emit light. There is an aura that is emitted by rocks. Of course many rocks, especially crystals, are living entities. The light (or aura) that is emitted from crystals is magnificent.

Light is also emitted from foods. A marvelous book by David Wolfe entitled "Eating for Beauty" has page after page of pictures which display the light that food emanates. When food is alive, the light that is emanated is glorious, magnificent and astonishing.

The light that is emanated by food that is dead is pretty inconsequential. It is of course present, but you do not see many colors. You do not see a brilliant, strong illumination from dead foods. The light emitted is faint and dull.

Extend your awareness, then, to all living objects. There are some videos that are readily available on the internet that show what happens to plants when music is played. Plants actually dance just as humans dance when they hear music that is pleasing to them. When you track the auras that are emanated by plants in such circumstances you see a magnificent light show:

- *The light expands.*
- *The light contracts.*
- *The light shines brilliantly.*
- *The light dims proudly.*
- *The light emits colors that are brilliant.*

One fascinating guest on my radio show (the Parkinsons Recovery Radio Show) is Johan Boswinkel. He invented a biofeedback machine that measures the light that is emanated through the various meridians in the body. He explains that it really is a very low level of light, something equivalent to a candle at a distance of about 20 miles. We are not seeing a strong brilliant rays of light beam out of the body as you might see from the sunshine. Light, however, does come from within all cells of our body.

Johan uses his new invention which draws on the technology of Biophotonics to measure distortions in the light through the body. If the light is straight there is no distortion. If it is distorted, there is an imbalance. Using his device he determines the source of imbalances in the body. These distortions are the source of illness and disease.

For chronic conditions such as Parkinson's, he finds the source of the neurological problem is oftentimes the liver, the gall bladder or even an infected appendix - sources that most practitioners do not even consider.

We are all light bodies. Individuals who are users of street drugs such as cocaine or heroin or even more harmful substances emit a very dark energy from around their nose or from around their mouth. For police officers who are able to see auras, there is no mystery about who is addicted and who is not. All they have to do is look at an individual's aura. They can see dark energy hanging around that person's mouth or the person's nose.

A lot of information comes from the color of light that is emanated from bodies and the distance that it radiates from the body. Many people have the idea that auras are stagnant. They presumably hang two to three feet distant from the body.

Light that shines from the body is not stagnant. Auras are also not static. They are always shifting and changing. They are continuously expanding and contracting as a reflection of the life force and the pure essence that is emanating from the person.

If you are interested in actually being able to see auras - and I know some of you already see them as a matter of routine and habit - let me just suggest that you not look

16

directly at the person's body. Rather, look an inch or two above their head. The other important lesson to learn is not to try and grab the light that is emanated from the body you are observing. Do not go after it. Allow the light to come to you.

Just sit. Quiet your mind. Allow a couple of minutes to pass. Oftentimes you want to make sure that you are looking at a person who has given you permission or a person at a distance that will not be upset by the fact that you are staring at them.

Every human being emits light. There are now instruments that measure that. You can get readings of your aura if you would like from photographers who have special equipment. We are all light beings.

Consider giving yourself the fascinating challenge of beginning to track the auras of plants, food, and other individuals. You will be mysteriously engaged as you see brilliant colors of light emanating from a person's head and from their heart. When a person is excited about what they are doing they exude the most magnificent color of purple that defies description.

Enjoy yourself as you continue to honor and acknowledge the presence of light in your life whether the source of that light is:

- *The sun.*
- *Headlights on a car.*
- *Light bulbs in your house.*
- *Live food*
- *Plants that dance to music.*
- *Individuals that you love who exude joyful,
  gorgeous rays of gold light.*

Enjoy yourself thoroughly as you acknowledge the
authentic source of light. We are all light beings.

Exercise Three: Notice Trees

My simple yet profound invitation is to take close and careful notice of trees.

- *What is their shape?*
- *Are they tall?*
- *Are they short?*
- *Are they fat?*
- *Are they skinny?*
- *Is the tree you happen to be noticing in the moment shaggy?*
- *Is it sculptured in shape much like a Christmas tree?*
- *What is the height of the tree that your eyes now gaze on?*

Notice the branching. Notice in particular the color of the tree, the color of the leaves, the color of the bark and the texture of the bark. Notice the type of foliage that emanates from the trunk of this most magnificent tree that you chose to gaze at.

Of course you can't inspect each tree that you see with any great detail. Perhaps you might spend some time sitting under a tree doing just that. As you walk and as you drive however, devote your attention to taking quite

19

seriously the challenge of taking in the magnificence of the trees that you pass by. They exude a life force of immense power.

In some cases becoming mindful of trees will be a fleeting notice at best. In other situations - perhaps on a walk - invite yourself:

1. **to stop**
2. **to turn**
3. **to look**
4. **to take in**

The most magnificent presence of the tree that happens to call out to you in the moment.

If you live in an area where there are few tall and magnificent trees – perhaps a desert - choose to observe sagebrush or grass or bushes instead of trees. Trees are not required.

Whether your focus is on trees or sagebrush - take their full essence in. Notice them with your eyes, ears and nose. Trees are a miracle on earth that we take for granted.

- Reverse the habit of taking trees for granted.
- Acknowledge their magnificence and their divinity.

After all, we share the sacred space of the earth side by side along with them.

Deeper Meaning Behind Noticing Trees

My simple yet profound invitation was to take close and careful notice of trees. Whether your focus is on trees or sagebrush - take their full essence in. Notice them with your eyes, ears and nose. Trees are a miracle on earth that we take for granted. They are alive too. Frees feed us with oxygen. Without trees, we would not be alive today. We depend on one another to sustain life.

Exercise Four: Notice Red

This mindfulness challenge involves noticing the color red. Some mindfulness gurus take students who are blindfolded into a room they have never seen before. They remove the blindfold and ask the student to gaze around the room with the expectation that they will be asked to describe what is in the room. They are only given about 15 seconds. The blindfold is re-affixed and the question is asked,

> *"Now describe what is in this room."*

This is a particularly challenging task for most people. The task I have this week is nothing as difficult or onerous as that task, but in a way it has the same intent. The task is each day, throughout the entire week, to take notice of everything that has red or is the color red.

- *This might be red on a billboard, red on the highway, red on a signal light or a traffic sign.*
- *It may be red that you notice in a picture on a wall.*
- *It may be red in a carpet that you are walking on.*
- *It may be the texture of red on the walls of a room that you are entering or red that is worn by people who you encounter.*

Of course you might acknowledge red that you may yourself be wearing that day. You will soon know better than most people that red is found all over the place.

The task however is to take special notice every time you encounter the color red no matter where you find it. I invite you to let red find you. Consider this to be a serious search everyday as you meticulously search for red everywhere in the environment you find yourself in.

An ancillary assignment that you may want to undertake one or two or all seven days of the week is to keep a mental count of the number of times you spotted the color red. Don't actually make a record on a piece of paper or a notebook. See if you can remember the last number in the count and then add to that number when you see an object with the color red. Continue the count until you actually reach the number 100. If you get the end of the day and realize you are only at 64, do a meticulous search to find more and more objects that have the color red unit you reach the magical number of 100.

There is a final mindfulness invitation. This one is only for situations where you are in a secure, safe place. Do not consider doing this while driving or certainly not while operating heavy equipment machinery. When you are in a safe place and you spot the color red no matter what it happens to be on or where it is coming from - whether from the sky or the earth - something in nature or something man-made – allow yourself to receive and be soaked with the frequency of red. Allow yourself to become red each time that you see it.

Enjoy the experience as you encounter object after object that contains the color red. Marvel at the redness that you encounter.

Deeper Meaning Behind the Color Red

Before I explain the significance of noticing the color red, I invite you to reflect back on the last four days and ask yourself:

1. *Did you take on the assignment to notice red?*
2. *How frequently did you mindfully pay attention to your environment so that you could detect red in every object you encountered?*

Did you perhaps get the assignment and although you intended to take it seriously, the task somehow was forgotten. Life got in the way. You never encountered anything red; or if you did, you didn't notice.

Make a mental note of the extent to which you undertook this assignment seriously.

© Parkinsons Recovery

- *Did you count the number of times every day in your head that you encountered red?*
- *Did you reach the number 100 and quit or did you keep counting?*
- *On some days did you just not want to do it because it was too hard or too mentally challenging even though making a mental count creates new neural networks?*

Reflect back on the past few days and acknowledge your approach to the challenge of noticing the color red.

Let me now explain the significance of this challenge. In one way it comes across as a childlike game, something like Waldo. Waldo is an entity that is found in children's pictures. The child has to look all over the picture before they find Waldo. When they spot him they point and say, "Hooray!." The parent of course also says "Yes!" But actually, the assignment to find red has far more serious and important implications than simply a child's game – although we don't want to underestimate the importance of that as well.

Colors are associated with frequencies. Frequencies are imbedded in our energy field. Individuals with Parkinson's tend to have energy that surrounds the upper part of their body. This of course is not true for all persons with Parkinson's but in general individuals who tend to encounter symptoms of Parkinson's are go getters.

- **They are focused.**
- **They are accomplished.**
- **They make things happen.**
- **They are the go-to people of the world.**

If we didn't have that kind of energy not much would be accomplished in any country or any culture. It is a wonderful, marvelous, delicious, delightful energy that makes things happen. This also has implications for how an individual with the go-to energy runs the frequencies around their physical body.

The energy for many persons with Parkinson's tends to be the colors that you find over on the right-side of a rainbow, perhaps purple, gold or blue; but not the lower frequency colors. The lowest frequency in the human energy field is red. It is associated with the first chakra. That is the energy input to the human body that enters between our two legs.

A chakra looks like a funnel of sorts, almost like a tornado. The tip of the cone is nested up against the coccyx or the bottom of the spine. We all have first chakras.

The more we are able to connect with the color red, the more we are able to strengthen, enlarge and nourish that particular chakra so that we are more solidly connected with mother earth. When our first chakras are open and vibrant, we centered and balanced.

Connecting with the color red helps mobility problems. Why? It addresses the center of balance. We are connected to the earth when we are solidly receiving and connected to the color red. The color red is not just a cool color that you find in a child's box of crayons. Red is a very specific frequency. It is the frequency that is associated with allowing us to be physically present to ourselves and to others.

This notion is called "grounding." It means that instead of feeling like we are unstable at the top of our bodies (and in our heads) as we have difficulty walking, we are solid. We are able to step with the right foot, then the left foot with assurance and grace and poise. We anchor ourselves into the core of the earth. There is little chance of falling when our first chakras are open and balanced.

How do you make sure that your first chakra is open, strong and vibrant? One easy way is to connect with the color red. This is not a mental issue however. You have to allow the color red to essentially soak into your body. You have to "feel" the color red. Once you do, the first chakra opens up magnificently. You do not have to force it open. It happens effortlessly.

Continue throughout the rest of the week to notice the color red. Every time you spot red, allow yourself to resonate with that color. When you do, you literally are connecting with the frequency that nourishes and strengthens your first chakra. The work you are doing this week is obtaining relief from symptoms using your own self-administered color therapy treatments. No color therapist is needed this week!

This mindfulness challenge is particularly useful to anyone who might be having mobility challenges or balance challenges. No medications are needed here. This is something you can do for yourself throughout the day. Resonating with the frequency of red means that balance can no longer be a problem because you are anchored to mother earth. Mother earth will not allow you to fall or stumble or freeze when you are connected to it.

Enjoy encountering the color red the rest of the week.

- *Become red.*
- *Be red.*
- *Feel red.*
- *Resonate with red.*

If you are fighting against doing this it probably means that this is an exercise you need to take very seriously. As you think back to the question I asked in the very beginning - to what extent did you engage this exercise seriously - if you did not, it may be that now is a good time to hunker down and to take it more seriously; to reach that count of 100 and furthermore, each time you encounter anything, whether in nature, the sky, the earth, a person, an object, a food is red, stop and resonate with that color.

When you do encounter red it can have marvelous and magnificent healing consequences. And, by the way, it is a free healing each time. This doesn't cost anything. You are helping your body to come back into full balance. Isn't that cool?

Exercise Five: Notice Yellow

This mindfulness challenge invites you to take in and notice the color yellow wherever you go and wherever you are. Wherever you go, make a count of everything yellow that you encounter, just as you did with the color red.

If you see a plant that has yellow in it, count that as one. If you see cars, plates, pictures, carpets, houses or any objects anywhere that contain yellow count them. Make a mental tally throughout the day. When you reach the count of 100, you can stop if you so choose or you can keep counting.

Keeping a mental count of the number of yellow things and objects and entities and clothes and objects that you have noticed is a straightforward way of forging new neural networks. You create new neural networks and nourish your neurological system even when you forget the count!

To summarize, this week the focus is on the color yellow. As you now know, when you focus on yellow you are also resonating with the frequency of yellow.

Deeper Implications Behind the Color Yellow

I am quite sure you have been pondering the deeper meaning behind spending your time counting everything yellow that you encounter; what a silly activity to engage in, especially for an adult. My invitation for reflection is the following.

You have had a couple of weeks break from noticing the color red. What difference have you observed in how you approached and engaged this assignment – that is the challenge to notice the color yellow – when contrasted with the assignment several weeks ago which was to notice the color red?

Did you accept this assignment more willingly? Were you more dedicated to keeping the count each day? Did you reach the count of 100 each day when you were counting yellow?

In contrast, when counting red did you find some days that you literally did not notice anything red? Did you notice with the challenge to notice red that you encountered some hesitation, some resistance, some distaste for that assignment whereas the assignment this week (the assignment to notice the color yellow) seemed to go more smoothly?

Part of the reason the challenge this week might have been easier may be that you had some practice doing it. There is another reason altogether you might have experienced a difference.

Yellow as a frequency is a mental frequency. It is the frequency we resonate at when we are engaged in mental activity. As I am creating this mindfulness exercise to notice the color yellow, I am resonating at the equivalent frequency of yellow. I am on what we call the mental level.

Many individuals who currently experience symptoms of Parkinson's tend to remain on the yellow frequency wave band. They engage a great deal of thinking throughout each minute of the day. Many of these thoughts are not in their best and highest good. It helps, then, to switch off the volume on the mental level which opens the door to allowing other delicious states of awareness to unfold.

Of course resonating at the mental level (the equivalent frequency of yellow) is the reason for prior successes and victories. It is a gift. It is a skill to have strengthened this particular level of the human energy field.

It is also important, however, to balance our energy field out.

- Acknowledge the role of all the levels (and frequencies) including red, which is that grounding

32

level that helps stabilize our mobility and our intention to recover fully and completely.

- Acknowledge now any difference you might have noticed between doing the two assignments; between noticing yellow and red.
- Acknowledge that health and wellness is a function of balance - of being able to absorb the color red and the color yellow in balanced doses.

There is absolutely nothing wrong with being mental. It certainly benefited me throughout my entire life. The disadvantage of living a life solely on the mental level is when that is the only frequency level we tend to operate on, when that is the frequency we are always resonating at,

- **We do not feel our feelings.**
- **We do not feel connected to Mother Earth.**
- **We are not deeply connected to others.**
- **We isolate ourselves.**
- **We withdraw and literally wither away.**

Living life in constant fear can be a consequence. Becoming anxious about each new challenge in life can become a habit.

To maintain a vibrant energy field that entails all chakras open and all meridians cleared, it is important to resonate with frequencies at all levels of the energy field. There are many frequencies of course. Here we are only talking about two levels of the field (or two frequencies) - the ones specifically associated with the colors yellow and red.

Enjoy the rest of the week as you continue to notice yellow. If you want to be ambitious, continue to notice red also. If in fact you notice now that it is a little easier to find yellow than it is to find red, I assure you it is not because there is a deficiency of the color red in the world. It really is all about resisting being connected with that grounding frequency of red in favor of the mental frequency which is equivalent to the color yellow.

May you have a delightful time the rest of the week as you continue to even out the resonances of frequencies throughout your human energy field and become mindful of the value of resonating at all frequencies. With greater mindfulness your journey down the road to **recovery will become** effortless.

Exercise Six: Notice Blue

The mindfulness challenge this week is to become a detective wherever you happen to find yourself – whether it is inside a familiar room or outside in a place you have never visited - to notice and acknowledge the color blue wherever you encounter it.

By a detective I mean the following. As you move from one place to the next, focus your attention on searching for the color blue. Anything counts—pictures, carpets, leafs, flowers, hairs of people that have been colored blue, cars, buildings, products in stores, clothes, lipstick, the sky, crayons, food... Maintain a watchful gaze wherever you find yourself. Acknowledge and notice the color blue.

A companion challenge (if you decide to accept the challenge to notice the color blue) is to keep a count of the number of objects that contain blue throughout the week. Each day, begin the count with the number one and increment the count with each new object that you find which contains blue. Don't count on a piece of paper. Count in your mind.

What in the world is the reason for keeping a count in your mind each day? It forges new neural networks. If you forget the count at 1:30 in the afternoon and think to yourself,

> *"Oh my gosh, I can't believe I can't remember the count from earlier today."*

Do not worry or fret about it. The effort of simply trying to keep count actually works just as well in creating new neural networks. It is engaging the effort of trying that makes the difference.

By the end of the day you will have a total count to acknowledge as you close your eyes for bed. Whatever that final tally may be - whether 24, 82, 109 or 1,022 - close your eyes and celebrate your success with keeping count from the beginning to the end of the day. Acknowledge the beauty and wonders of the world as it is exhibited through the magnificent color of blue.

Deeper Meaning Behind Noticing Blue

I am quite sure that you are wondering

> *"What in the world is the underlying meaning behind the little simple task of noticing the color blue. First red. Then yellow. Now blue?"*

This particular task allows each of us who engage this mindfulness exercise to turn off the switch and the unhealthy program of negative thoughts that happens to be running inside our minds. Most of us have a program that continuously runs second after second; we are always churning the same worrisome thoughts, the same concerns. We find that we are nurturing stress because we simply can't change the channel of churning out negative thoughts. We cannot find a way to switch to another channel. How in the world do we do tune into a different channel?

Some people simply try to stop thinking unhealthy thoughts. There is little doubt which thoughts are healthy and which thoughts are not. This strategy can work for a few seconds but usually the thoughts will immediately creep back in. An easier way – and I might add a more fruitful and enjoyable way – is to literally switch into an entirely different program that is not only unfamiliar, but quite simple to do.

The program this week is to notice the color blue. It switches the program that you habitually run over and over in your mind. Instead of churning the very same concerns and thoughts and worries that are promulgating stress throughout all the tissues of your body, you literally switch that program off. It is as if you are a computer and you are saying to yourself,

> *"This program is not going to be running today. Today we're going to be turning on a different program to run our thoughts."*

The program that you turn on turns out to be a harmless – and I might add somewhat mindless program – of noticing a very specific color. In this case, the magnificent color of blue. Becoming mindful of a very specific color will do just that. It switches off one program that is creating problems and turns on another program that is positive, interesting, enjoyable, fun and energizing.

There is another important reason why blue has a magnificent value to each of us. The fifth chakra is located in the throat. It supports and nurtures our voice. The equivalent color of the fifth chakra turns out to be blue. When I say equivalent color I am also talking about the frequency that is associated with the throat and fifth chakra.

Some people with Parkinson's confront challenges with vocalization—with being able to talk clearly and coherently. Noticing the color blue is an indirect way of healing a chakra at the fifth level (which spins at the center of the throat). When problems with vocalization occur, the fifth chakra spins erratically and chaotically. If the spin is not wide and smooth, the organs associated with the throat do not function properly.

When you connect with the color blue you resonate with the frequency that is the equivalent of the color blue. In so doing, you entrain that fifth chakra to stop the wobbling, to stop the skirting from side to side and to enact an even, smooth and nurturing movement that circles around

© Parkinsons Recovery

evenly and gently so that your voice can be heard loudly and clearly. The color blue is healing for just this reason.

As you were searching for blue these past few days you were also connecting and resonating with the equivalent frequency of blue. You were nurturing your fifth chakra back to full health and wellness.

Have you noticed that your ability to speak has been enhanced as you have been the detective on the search for the color blue? That is why. Oftentimes an innocent task can yield enormous dividends and returns.

Have fun as you continue to be a detective searching everywhere you encounter for the color blue. You have the potential of achieving two important outcomes: nurturing thoughts that are good for your health and healing a voice that can be heard by all.

Parkinsons Recovery Programs

Has your work on these exercises been stress free? Has it been helpful in reducing your symptoms? I certainly hope so! This is the primary reason I developed the mindfulness exercises in the first place.

If you struggled with pacing out these mindfulness exercises so as not to induce more stress, there are several Parkinsons Recovery programs that might help expedite your recovery. My Parkinsons Recovery Mindfulness Program sends the mindfulness exercises in an email to you each and every week. The initial exercise is sent to your email address on day one of the week and the deeper implications are sent four days later. The Parkinsons Recovery Mindfulness Program takes one full year to complete as each exercise is introduced one week at a time. For more information visit:

www.stress.parkinsonsrecovery.com

Parkinsons Recovery Memberships involve a variety of support websites that are essential to recovery. A difference mindfulness exercise is posted each week. For more information on Parkinsons Recovery memberships visit:

www.parkinsonsrecovery.org

Of course, the approach that works for many people is to purchase a single volume of the Parkinsons Recovery Mindfulness program at a time as you have already done! See the introduction for a listing of all nine Parkinsons Recovery Mindfulness volumes.

Thank you for Your Support

On behalf of the thousands of followers of Parkinsons Recovery, I want to thank you for your purchase of this booklet. One hundred percent (100%) of the profits purchases of my books and programs help subsidize the many free services I offer through Parkinsons Recovery -

www.parkinsonsrecovery.com

For information about other products, services and programs visit -

www.parkinsonsrecovery.me

www.ingramcontent.com/pod-product-compliance
Lightning Source LLC
Chambersburg PA
CBHW070236290526
45789CB00004B/1653

* 9 7 8 1 5 0 2 3 2 1 1 1 4 *